Swimming the Seasons

A Freshwater Almanac

IN THE MOMENT

Polly Atkin

Saraband

Published by Saraband
3 Clairmont Gardens
Glasgow, G3 7LW
www.saraband.net

ISBN: 9781916812383

Printed and bound in Great Britain by Clays Ltd, Elcograf S.p.A.

1 2 3 4 5 6 7 8 9

MIX
Paper | Supporting responsible forestry
FSC® C018072

WINNER: Lakeland Book of the Year 2024, for *Some of Us Just Fall*

LONGLISTED: Wainwright Prize for Nature Writing 2024 and 2025

Praise for The Company of Owls

"Beautifully written and densely observant ... There is much food for thought in this wonderful and wholly original book." —*Mail on Sunday*

"This touching, gentle offering shows that, given a humble heart and willingness to stand still in Nature and look and listen, you can get closer to owls than you'd imagine." —*Country Life*

Praise for Some of Us Just Fall

"A timely, lyrical and insightful exploration of the stories we tell about our bodies … her descriptions of her daily walks and swims were so beautiful." —*The Times*

"With a poet's insight and a deep understanding of place, Atkin pulls us again and again to witness ... I was immersed." —Katie Hale

Praise for Recovering Dorothy

"Polly Atkin argues for Dorothy's place in the writing of illness … A narrowing world, she reminds us, need not lead to a narrowing of the self." —*The Guardian*

"A timely reappraisal … told with great sensitivity and … a grounded perspective of Dorothy's everyday life in the Lakeland landscape." —*Cumbria Life, Book of the Month*

Also by Polly Atkin

Narrative non-fiction

The Company of Owls

Some of Us Just Fall:
On Nature and Not Gettinwg Better

Recovering Dorothy:
The Hidden Life of Dorothy Wordsworth

Poetry

Emergency Dream

Much With Body

Basic Nest Architecture

Contents

Water is a portal. It invites us to think about time differently. Its surfaces reflect migration and movement and cultural change.

—Alycia Pirmohamed, *rivering*

Getting In

This book is neither a guide nor a diary. It is not a map to follow, though you can follow it and me as I swim through a year of the seasons in the lakes and rivers of the English Lake District. It is a record of swims past that holds within it the promise of swims future. It is a record of particular swims in particular places in my particular body, but in its particularity, you may find space to place yourself, your body, your memories, your rivers, your lakes, your hopes, your plans. It springs from the waters of Lakeland, where I have lived for the best part of twenty years, but like all water, it carries memories and potential from far beyond this north-westerly outjutting of England. I hope it can bring you a little of the joy I find in swimming, wherever you are, and however you meet it.

Though it is not a guide and does not seek to tell you how or where to swim, in sharing how and where I swim, I hope there is something in it to learn from, whether you are a swimmer yourself or are reading about it from a safe, dry distance.

To swim is an act of attention, to the self, and to everything beyond the self. To what moves between them. To those who share the water with you – human and nonhuman – and to the water itself. The lake is a mirror in which to see yourself and see your place in the world, to see the place that is your world thrown back at you from a different perspective.

To swim through the seasons is a practice of ongoing learning – about yourself and the world around you. About your environment and your responses to your environment. About how you want to relate to the world and to other living beings.

Swimming is repetition, stroke after stroke after stroke. It can become a kind of meditation. But this repetition moves you. You move yourself forward by doing the same thing, over and over again. The way I swim outdoors extends this exercise in repetition. My swimming year is a process of returning and returning to the same spot or spots, finding something different and something same. It is a layering of memory and time. I do the same thing again and again with intention and attention and I move forward. I move forward with an ease I do not know out of the water. This is what swimming is to me, what it gives me.

To know how to swim, you need to know why you swim, what you want to get from it. You need to know what you are seeking when you go to the water. Exertion or relaxation, companionship or solitude, excitement or calm, peril or comfort. Immersion in the other, or restoration to the self.

The reasons I swim and the things I value in it may not apply to you. I can tell you about why I swim, and how that informs how I swim, but I cannot tell you how to do it, or what might matter about it for you. You can only work that out for yourself.

You also need to know what you don't want to get from swimming. Some people swim to remember their body; to find mindfulness in the shock of embodiment. I do not need to be reminded of embodiment. I live with chronic incurable illness, which means my body is a noisy companion, always making itself felt and heard. I swim not to forget my body, but to let it forget for a little while how hard it has to work to do small things that many people take for granted. I swim to release my body from gravity, to let it let go of all the strain of keeping itself piled one bone on top of another.

But my conditions can also make it difficult to swim, especially outdoors in ever-changing environments and conditions. I can't walk far, especially carrying kit, so most swim-walks are out of bounds for me. I need to know I can get in and out of the water easily, without injuring myself. I am prone to infection, so I am careful about when I swim as well as where. I cannot be blasé about cyanobacteria blooms or sewage leaks. My conditions are energy-limiting, and can turn quickly. I cannot push myself beyond my limits in the water or getting to the water and expect to be able to get myself home safely too. I can't expect to be able to swim every day, and sometimes I can't swim at all. If I do swim several days in a row, I can expect to be too tired to do anything else.

Like many chronically ill people, I live in a state of discomfort. I don't need any more of it, or to be reminded peril exists. Peril is a constant companion, just as pain is. I swim in ways that seek to optimise my enjoyment whilst avoiding making anything worse. It is often said the benefits of cold water swimming come through exposure to acceptable risk, but everything seems such a risk to me there is nothing distinctive or enthralling about the idea of it, not for my mind nor my body. I swim in ways calculated to minimise risk as far as I can, not court it. In many ways, I am a living mirror image of the idealised wild swimmer.

The hardest part to explain to people is this. I swim all year round outdoors in this northern mountainous region, but I do not like the cold. Nothing about the cold brings me pleasure. I get no thrill from it, no hint of the fabled cold rush that draws swimmers back and back to the cold. I am always cold, and in winter, it gets deep into my bones and I cannot dislodge it. If I get cold, I cannot get warm again. I have poor circulation in my extremities, and they are almost always cold. Cold hands, cold feet, cold nose. It takes a lot to warm them up. On any given day in winter, you will find me working tucked up in a thick blanket with a hot-water bottle just to thaw enough to begin to think. I know swimmers with the same connective tissue disorder I have who experience relief from their daily pain in cold water. It does not work like that for me. Cold water brings all my old injuries back to life, resurrecting the pain of old broken bones, and triggering excruciating muscle spasms. Why, then, do I choose to take all these cosy layers off even on the coldest of days, and get into cold water?

This is what I tell those who ask me that: I love to swim more than I hate being cold. I don't swim for sport. I don't really swim for exercise, although it is the least painful exercise my body knows. I swim for love. It is love that keeps me swimming all year round, despite the cold. I have always loved being in water. I love to be underwater. If I could breathe down there, I might stay there. Swimming is the closest thing to flying I know, the closest thing to extending beyond humanhood. What I am seeking when I swim is not bodily exertion but sensory immersion and extension. To me, swimming is transformation, transcendence – a kind of natural magic through which the extraordinary is revealed in the everyday, over and over again.

I swim to recognise my disabled body as just one body amongst many within the body of the water. I swim to share space with the other lives around me. I swim to spy on the heron from within the water, to watch the wagtail flit over chirruping, to meet dragonflies and damselflies eye to eye. And a huge part of this is beauty. I swim breaststroke for the most part not just to save my shoulders from the over-extension of crawl, but because I want to see everything around me as I swim. I want to see the fells and the sky and the trees on the shore reflected in the water, and I want to part them with my hands and draw them aside, fold them into the lake and into each other. That is the alchemy of swimming. I swim to watch the fells appear and disappear and appear and disappear in the scrying glass of the lake. I swim to fold myself through them, to see us as we are, different portions of the same matter.

I swim to see my body as it is. The way my limbs refracted through the water look how they so often feel – out of joint, distorted – how the water makes the invisible visible. A manifestation of pain made beautiful without making it neat, without fixing it.

I swim to see the way light moves on skin underwater, making it part of the movement of light and water, the interchange between them. The way moving light bounces from the moving surface of the water and projects its movement onto bodies on land: the trunks of trees, the limbs of a swimmer drying in the sun on the shore. Even out of the water, you are part of the water. I swim to remember this.

I cannot get enough of lake light. Of light through water, light from water. It is one of the most beautiful things in the world to me, and I want that beauty all year round. So it is that the lake on a clear, icy day in winter is so extraordinarily beautiful that I long to be in it more than I dread its cold. I want to be part of it, a body in its body, even if only for five minutes. I want to be part of the way it bends light. I want my pale winter-face like a small moon reflecting the light of the midwinter sun, and throwing it back down into the viscous water.

This is what I mean by love. This is why I swim.

There are many things I have learnt in the years I have swimming been all year round. The most useful are these:

- Only you can judge what your body can tolerate on any given day. No one else can tell you what conditions will be safe and pleasurable for you. Do not follow someone into a storm-swept lake or icebound stream or a cold waterfall just because they say it will be fine. The important thing is if it feels fine to you, and you know your own responses.
- What feels safe and pleasurable to you will alter with the conditions of your body as much as with the weather. It will change with how tired you are, how stressed, with your sleep patterns and hormones as much as with the seasons. You need to be alert to your body as it is on the day you take it to the water, not an idea of how it may be in general.
- Always make sure you know how you're going to get out of the water before you get in. This might sound obvious, but one of the most hilarious and alarming swims I have ever had was with a dear friend, also an experienced swimmer, in a river spot she had swum in before but in a different season, the level higher, and no nettles covering the banks as on the early September day we went there together. We did not stop to think as we dropped in off the muddy bank that I would

not be able to lift myself back out. When we realised, after we had swum for as long as we should safely have done, we began a frantic search along the bank for a spot that had a foothold or handhold, or where the river was shallower, or there was a rock or tree I could use as a step up. My friend, less responsive to nettle stings than me, heaved herself up onto the nettle-strewn bank as I tried out different spots for a good ten minutes, trying not to panic as I lost feeling in my hands and feet. Eventually, we found a place further down the bank on the opposite shore, where we could also return along a footpath without crashing through brambles and neck-high nettles in bikinis with far too much skin bared. We were weeping with laughter and relief by the time I was flopping around on the bank, covered in mud, like a fish drowning in air. But it could have had a very different ending, and served as a useful reminder. Always know your exit. Check it is accessible to you before you enter the water. Don't rely on knowledge from a previous swim, or from other swimmers.

› Remember that any swimming companions will have a different tolerance of heat and cold and exertion. Don't assume every body is the same as your body.

› Nothing bad is going to happen if you don't go for a swim.

› If you get to your chosen swim spot and you don't feel right, or the water doesn't, you can always go home again and not swim. Better no swim and safe than risking your own or anyone else's safety. Times I've turned home and not swum include days when I got to the lake and broken up sheets of ice were flying from the surface of the lake in a horizontal wind, like glass behind thrown through the air; days when I got to the lake and found someone's garden furniture floating past amongst other unseen storm debris; many days throughout the year when I've travelled to some river or other but found it too terrifyingly high after too much rain to even dip a toe in, or too low and stagnant after none. It is far better to wistfully long for a swim that could not take place than painfully regret one that shouldn't have.

› It should be enjoyable. If it's not, it might be time to rethink how, when and why you're swimming.

Getting In

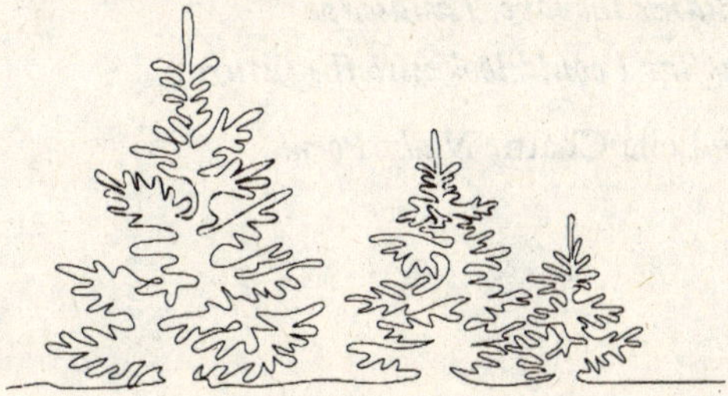

Blame the lake. Landscape
so flat I could look into the future

—Leila Chatti, *Night Poem*

Water Biosecurity

It seems obvious to me that if you swim somewhere you love, you should also look after it and out for it. That if a place gives you something, you should give something to it too. That a place that gives you joy should warrant your care. But I'm aware that's not obvious to everyone. We're primed to think about the impact of a place on our health, not necessarily the impact of our presence on a place's health. In the last decade, water, rebranded as 'blue space', has increasingly been valued not for its own sake, but for the mental, social and physical health benefits it may offer to humans – whether the blue mind state that is meant to offer an antidote to the woes of modern life, or the cold water rush that is meant to reset the body's inner workings.

Even if they want to be thoughtful, not everyone might not know what looking after a body of water and its inhabitants might mean, and it might look different for everyone. At its simplest, it can mean not disturbing wildlife, it can mean leaving no trace, and it can also mean taking nothing with you. That includes making sure you're not spreading invasive species or pollutants from body of water to body of water.

Everything you wear in the water should be carefully checked over, cleaned and dried between uses. Care should be taken to avoid rinsing any weed down the drain and so reintroducing it into the water system. The best advice is to rinse all kit in a bucket and pour the water out over hard ground or grass where it can drain without entering the water system, but that often seems like an impossible conundrum to me. When the ground is wet here, everything funnels down into the becks and the lake. The drains are overloaded at the best of times, and when a surge in visitor numbers coincides with a surge in rainfall, the whole system overflows. In the last few years, I've seen an increase in Himalayan balsam, skunk cabbage and Japanese knotweed on the shores of Grasmere and Rydal and the surrounding tarns, and an increase in waterweed.[1] Failing infrastructure and changes in human activity combine to make their spread seem inevitable, but it's not. We can always do better, try harder. We can fix what is broken, update crumbling systems, change practices and norms.

Biosecurity in our lakes is increasingly important as it is increasingly threatened, between climate change and the rise in popularity of watersports and eventing cultures that encourage people to travel to multiple lakes and tarns in a single day. All of our lakes and rivers are at continual risk and need more care and responsibility shown to them. Community groups do what they can – from litter-picking by groups like the Grasmere Wombles to water testing by groups like Ambleside Action for the Future – but we need a sea change in attitude, policy and funding to prioritise the wellbeing of our lakes and rivers over the wellbeing of human water users. There will be no calming blue mind state for any of us if the blue spaces themselves are dead or dying, unsafe to humans and nonhumans alike.

The high-profile Save Windermere campaign, initiated in 2021 by Matt Staniek to protect Windermere from pollution – pollution caused largely by failing infrastructure – has shown that it is possible turn awareness into action when the awareness is loud and national enough, though there is a lot of work ahead.[2]

Grasmere's history in the last half century shows that positive changes can happen when policy and infrastructure are attuned to a lake's needs. In the late 1990s it was Grasmere, not Windermere, that was making the news as 'in danger of dying of pollution'. Just as is happening in Windermere now, Grasmere was being poisoned by phosphate overload from failing sewage systems and farm run-off. In 1998, the campaigning of the Grasmere Residents

Clean Lake Group was reported as far afield as Melbourne, Australia. On 31st December 1999, under the headline '"Dead Lake" fears for Grasmere', The Westmorland Gazette recorded ongoing efforts in Grasmere to counter what the Environment Agency called 'thirty years of pollution from inadequate sewage treatment' that was destroying the ecology of the lake.[3] Long-serving Lake Parish councillor Vivienne Rees called for testing of the water, but the South Lakeland District Council's response was merely to 'discourage swimming in the lakes'. Testing was deemed too costly, the problems insurmountable. It was better just to keep people out of and away from the water. On the first day of the new millennium, the paper reported that North West Water had confirmed it would install a new pumping station, after 'solid matter [was] spotted floating in the water' as well as blue-green algae. All this will sound very familiar to anyone who has been following the current situation in Windermere.

Grasmere recovered. It was brought back from the brink of death by the tireless work of residents who cared about its wellbeing enough to fight for it for years. But it is always in precarious balance. It should be encouraging that change was made, but it was slow. The Lake Parish Council raised concerns in 1997, and it was 2003 before planning permission was passed for the new pumping station, and even then there were concerns about the quality of the work and how well it would serve the village's needs. At that time the lake was still being described as 'polluted and unsafe for children', the new sewage works only 'the beginning of a long journey to clean up the lake.'[4] In the years I've lived here, there have been continual problems with the sewers becoming blocked and overflowing, which contributed to the flood damage in the village during Storm Desmond in December 2015, and cause lesser problems in every heavy rainfall.

Anyone who pays attention to the health of our waterways will be familiar with the problem of storm overflow discharge and inadequate sewage works. In 2024, there were 115 sewage dumps into Grasmere recorded, lasting a total duration of 1,247 hours, equivalent to 1.73 months of sewage discharge over twelve months. In the same year, Windermere experienced over 6,300 hours of sewage overflow from six different sites, a reduction on the 2023 high of 8,787 – over a year's-worth of continual overflow. The Ambleside Action For A Future residents' group monitors Windermere's water quality, and weekly testing at Waterhead has found unacceptably high levels of E. coli and other bacteria in alarming frequency.

Twenty-five years ago in Grasmere, the SLDC's attempts to discourage swimming in the lake worked in part, or else the state of the lake itself did. When I moved here in 2006, older residents would warn us not to swim in the lake, that it wasn't safe. For the first two years I lived here, I almost never swam in Grasmere, sticking to the tarns and rivers. Only a few headstrong or foolish swimmers would brave Grasmere and its reputation as toxic soup. By the time I did start swimming in it regularly, the water quality had already improved dramatically, given the tools to maintain its own health. In recent decades, it has been one of the cleanest of the central lakes, but the current state of Windermere shows how fragile that balance is, and how much it relies on upkeep of perpetually underfunded infrastructure by companies and authorities that do not take their responsibilities seriously enough.

Those of us who spend time in and by water must do so responsibly, but we should all also be asking for more than this. We need a culture of care for water, a broader recognition of the central importance of clean water to all life.

Research conducted in 2024 by the Campaign for National Parks found that 'just 39 per cent of rivers and 15 per cent of lakes within [English] National Parks [are] in an ecologically healthy state.'[5]

Grasmere has not been judged above 'moderate' in its health. As they explain:

> Even in the most pristine rivers and lakes in England's National Parks, traces of toxic chemicals including mercury and other priority hazardous substances are found. Because of these toxic chemicals, which can remain in the ecosystem for decades, not a single water body in an English National Park is in good overall health.

We need to keep our lakes and rivers clean for their own sake, but doing so benefits everyone who lives in and by them, human and nonhuman. It benefits everyone who visits here. Anyone who has enjoyed in the Lake District owes those lakes and rivers care in return. If we do not deal with them fairly and responsibly, there will be nothing left to enjoy.

These, of course, were the moments when being alive was enough. Swimming, bread and marmalade, sitting high in a beech tree in the golden eye of the morning sun – that was life. One flew then, like a gay ship with the wind in its sails, over the cold black bottomless waters of misgiving.
—Rose Macaulay, *Dangerous Ages*

May

bluebells – dragonflies – owlets

May is a month of magic, of metamorphosis. Sometimes May begins with snow. Snow on daffodils nodding on the lake shore. Snow with a 9.30pm sunset confusing all sense of time. The next week, sunburn, and bluebells – first a sole blue spear in a sheltered spot in the woods, then one in a sunny corner by the water, then more, more, more each day until everything is bluebells. The woods and fells a blueish haze, the air sweet with them. Everything seems filtered through the blue-violet-lilac blur of the bluebells, the light itself blueish, as though emanating from them, or off them.

Each day, the light gets longer and longer, the lake warmer, the woods louder with new life and song. The promise of the summer to come grows within the shifting festival of Bluebell Season. Everything is buzzing, growing, singing. Anything is possible in May, and May makes everything seem possible.

Magnolia blooms against the blue sky, pied flycatchers returning to the woods after their long commute, tawny owlets leaving their nests to explore the rustling, scented world. At the house, lily-of-the-valley coming into flower amongst the columbines and yellow poppies, then the blousy old pink roses around the door. They don't last long, the roses, but they smell amazing. The last of the roe deer have shed the velvet from their antlers. I see them in the evenings stepping delicately amongst the flag irises and cuckoo flowers. The martins and swallows return, one by one at first, then, like the bluebells, many.

The lake has its own blue explosion. Electric cyan damselflies cling to the reeds and skim the surface of the water, moving in clouds. Like the bluebells, they seem to reflect or refract light, making the blue air bluer. When you swim in May, you are swimming into the sweetening blue of the bluebell sky. Damselflies scatter around you, rest on your hair and shoulders. You are part of the blue.

The birches and beeches by the water's edge glow with the acid green of new leaf. I forget every year how muted and bare the spring is until they arrive, uncurling and stretching into space as if from a deep sleep inside the cave of the tree. Each afternoon I walk to the lake, there is more green catching the sun between the water and the road, less lake between the leaves. The copper beeches are already pinkening, and the bracken uncurling and reaching frondly for sky. By the end of the month, it will have swallowed the less-trodden paths and they will be closed to me till autumn.

Before I swam through all the seasons, May would be the beginning of my lake-swimming year. The first warm days that made me want to shed layers and seek the coolness I usually shrank from. I still think at this time of year of my first May living in the lakes, the second after I moved north. Of a swim in Buttermere mid-month with a group from the university I was studying at. The clarity of the water. The vision of academia I was given by the course leader stripping down to her swimming costume and leading the willing into the water. How in its cold depths I understood my floating body as barely breaking the surface of something vast and beautiful. How this could be a way to live. It feels a very long time ago now, but that swim set something in motion in me, was part of directing me towards the life I live now.

On the little beach I prefer to swim from, the sun lingers until after 7.30pm in the first week of the month, before it dips behind Silver Howe. It creeps away from the beach first, then the woods, then the fellside on the east of the valley. If I leave when it leaves the beach, I can cut through the woods to the high old road and walk all the way home in sun.

By the end of the second week, it is 8pm. It gets harder to leave the lake as the sun stays longer. I take a book, but half the time I just sit and watch the water, delighting in the little herds of squeaking ducklings who come by to visit; in being able to just dry like this in the sun.

With each week, I shed a layer of winter's insulation in the water. First socks, then gloves. One day, I might have my first bare-legged swim of the season, accompanied by ducklings, oystercatchers, a heron flying over.

The first lake swim of the year with hands bare in the water, without the pain of too-cold water, feels so exquisite, I keep turning the water over and over in my palms. Then maybe mid-month, maybe a little later, there will come a day that is mild and still enough, the water gentle and welcoming enough, that I realise I don't need my neoprene top to protect my neck and shoulders anymore. I walk into the water in my swimming costume, not shivering, barely a goosebump once I get moving. The few damselflies are hovering over the water, floating perpendicular to the reeds. The surface of the water is broken by fish jumping up to eat mayflies, which are everywhere. There are woodpeckers in the trees and wagtails strutting along the shore. My strokes lengthen and slow as the water warms, and the time I spend in the water lengthens too.

One day, I will walk into the lake, and once I have checked the level of cold against my hands, I will dive under for the first time that year, resurfacing several metres out, shaking droplets from my head, like the mergansers that patrol the lake.

I swim parallel to shore, loitering by the reedbeds to watch the damselflies, then, when they emerge, the dragonflies.

In May 2025, there were more dragonflies than I'd ever seen before, and every evening they circled me as I swam, buzzing past me, stopping mid-flight and reversing towards me to appraise me. Every swim, surrounded by dragonflies, green as the new leaves. We had almost three weeks without rain in May 2025, little wind on the water. Each evening, the lake was still and shining, the greening fells reflected in it perfectly, moving in and out of the sky as I moved through the water. After such a cold, wet year before, it felt like actual magic. Like I'd tumbled into another dimension.

By the end of the month, the makeover is complete. The trees are all in full leaf. Butterflies rest on the rocks on the shore in the sun, and the sun lasts so long into the evening it is hard to go home. Summer is almost here.

What a luxury to bathe now! It is gloriously hot, — the first of this weather. I cannot get wet enough. I must let the water soak into me. When you come out, it is rapidly dried on you or absorbed into your body, and you want to go in again. I begin to inhabit the planet, and see how I may be naturalised at last.

—Henry David Thoreau, *Journal* (1854)

June

foxgloves – froglets – sleepy fawns

In June, the light lasts forever in the lakes. You can finish a day's work and still have hours of daylight to enjoy. It barely gets dark, not truly dark. Twilight starts around ten. By midnight, it is dark enough to reveal the stars, but by two, they are fading into dawn already.

Time stretches out and swims stretch into it.

This time of long light and mild water before the heave and noise of the school holidays is precious. Everything is green – green everywhere so bright in the sun you can't look at it straight on. The green of the trees reflecting in the mirror of the lake is dazzling. Sun split through the profusion of leaves casts a glaze of enchantment over everything. On days like this, you can find a spotted roe deer fawn curled up and sleeping in the long grass right in the middle of a path you walk down weekly, badgers gambolling on a hill at golden hour. The bluebells have gone over and the verges are all long tapers of foxgloves, each one with a bee in it. The lanes buzz and chitter. There is an abundance to June, but a calm in it. There is so much time to be excessive in, there is no rush in the overflow.

At the lake, I swim alongside huge green dragonflies, and families of grey wagtails, who swoop into shore over my head once I've left it, and forage in the shallows in a row. From the water, I watch families of nuthatches move through the trees, goldcrests flitting from branch to branch, the woodpecker terrorising the other birds as usual.

In the long bright evenings, I don't want to go home to the dim indoors. Dinner time gets later and later. I walk home through the woods after nine, watched from the trees by tawny owlets, all silence and stares, and nestfuls of fledged flycatchers, trilling and hopping, and the opal gleam of the midsummer moon rising.

Rain comes, and with it, tiny froglets and toadlets who wriggle in under our front door and get stuck in the mud of our worn-out carpets. These days, I have to check the living room and hallway for froglets before bed, to release them from the hostile environment of the house. They arrive every year around this time, dispersing from the tarns where they spawn in the spring. They have a set route they want to follow, and they do not seem to care that our house is in their way. They want to come in the front door and out through the back. I've watched them do this every summer. The first year, it took me by surprise and I took it as a fluke. It was only when they returned the following summer that I began to understand our presence was disrupting their lives, not the other way round. One year, we found a fully grown frog halfway up the front door, just below the handle, as though after realising it was too large to squeeze under it, it was trying to open it instead. A few minutes more and it would have been hanging off the handle.

The house we have rented for the last decade was once home to labourers at Sykeside Farm. The two-storey slate building was saved from condemnation in the 1930s, and the doors and windows and layout we know date from that time. But there are ghosts of earlier doors, remnants of different lives. I don't know what greeted the annual distribution of froglets and toadlets before the doors we know, but I find it hard to believe they have been battling them every summer for the four centuries we are sure this building has stood here. Perhaps it was a byre below that the frogs and toads moved freely through, until it wasn't. Perhaps they come back every year hoping the way will be clear again. One day, they may inherit it all, but for now, I try and make sure none get stuck inside, at least.

Frogs and toads can breathe directly through their skin – a process called cutaneous respiration – frogs more readily than toads. Their thin and permeable skin is extraordinary – letting them breathe through long months of hibernation in the mud and drink without using their mouths – but it also makes them particularly sensitive to their environments, to extreme temperatures that dry out their skin and their homes, to pollution and toxins that enter straight into their bloodstream just as oxygen does.

June 2023 was the hottest I remembered here. Someone in the village said the beck behind their house hadn't been so dry since the legendary summer of 1976. The froglets and toadlets came late, when the rain did. In the cold non-summer of 2024, they did not come at all; only a couple arriving, confused, in the winter.

Tadpoles can pause their own metamorphosis into froglets depending on weather conditions or resources. They can wait out a year like this, staying in the form and place that makes most sense at the time, in the circumstances of the moment, where they can be safest, strongest. I think of this every June when they begin to appear in the house. They have chosen this as a good time to change. A good time to grow and explore. I see it as a condition of our tenancy to help them on their way.

As the froglets move through the house, at the lake, there are tadpoles swimming in the shallows amongst shoals of tiny fish, and the perch and trout scouting about when the lake bed falls away into the depths. We all do things in our own time.

Even in midsummer, the sun leaves our little north-facing garden by 5pm, and it's then that I put down my work and set out for the lake or a river knowing I have the long light evening ahead of me.

Long June evenings are made for river swimming, when the light skips through the water as it fizzes over the stones, for after-dinner swims when the heat has gone but the light lingers. Even a Cumbrian river is warm enough then to swoop under the surface, moving with the flow and the fish, swimming upstream against the rush of water to sit under a waterfall like a sprite. The stones retain the heat of the day even when the sun is gone, and will warm you as you dry.

I spent one midsummer night like this, a soft, sunlit evening when I swam towards the setting sun as it seemed to dive into the tumbling water, which held its light after it fell.

She got a pale green bathing-suit [...] Sometimes she put her bathing-dress on when she got up and didn't take it off until she went to bed – running down to the water for a plunge whenever she felt like it and sprawling on the sun-warm rocks to dry.

She had forgotten all the old humiliating things that used to come up against her in the night – the injustices and the disappointments. It was as if they had all happened to some other person.

—L.M. Montgomery, *The Blue Castle*

July

sundew – harebells – bilberries

All year, I wait for the luxurious swims of July, the days when it is warm enough to linger in the water, without moving even, to float on your back in the reflection of the sky. To dry out on the shore without changing. To swim again, because you're not too cold.

In July, I am living the dream of the green bathing suit – a swimming self I can put on in the morning and not take off till I get into bed. It's not always like this, of course, but if there is even a day or two of it, a few days in a row of heat when I swim every day, without once getting cold, if there is even a taste of that, it is enough.

July is real summer, peak summer. In the wood, the bilberries are ripening, and the wild raspberries, so you can graze, if you want, on the walk to and from the lake. Harebells bob on the banks of the rivers and the shore of the lake.

A few days of clear sun in July and the water is soft and mild. It is almost effortless to swim when the water is like this. You can skull across the smooth, shining surface like a giant, clumsy water boatman.

These are the days I swim across the lake – with friends or alone – and relax in the sunlit shallows on the far shore before swimming back, languorous and dreamy with contentedness. My stroke is long and relaxed; moves me with ease through the water. It takes so much less work for me to swim far further and longer than it does when the water is colder. Every year, I am tricked by this shift into thinking I am stronger, fitter, less fatigued. But in truth it is just that I am moving across the surface of the world with less friction, briefly.

If the summer has been fine, July should be the time to enjoy loitering in river pools at your leisure, but once the holidays start you might find yourself queuing for your turn like a walker trying to ascend Helvellyn on a bank holiday. Good weather brings many people, and I find my usual swimming spots occupied more often than not. I lurk in the reeds with the heron, both seeking a little pocket of quiet, sulking to find our accustomed territory shrunken.

From the lake, the world is all primary colours: bright green, bright blue, a big yellow sun. I turn it all over with my hands as I swim, feather one into the other. It is quietest the further from shore you are. I swim out in the middle of the lake to be alone, choosing my moment to dive under when between paddleboards passing.

As the holiday crowds grow, I seek quiet further afield, heading out when I can to the north or west of the county, avoiding hot spots like Wastwater, but choosing less-frequented river pools at anti-social times.

A colder July means fewer swimmers, so though the rivers and waterfalls are cold, they are all mine. My long-sleeved swimming costume comes back out, sometimes my neoprene top. I grumble about having to put a layer back on, but by the time I have swum back and forth under a packhorse bridge, water all glitter and bubble, or tried to reach the bottom of a deep pool beneath a shady waterfall, diving under and under without shivering too much, I am just pleased to be there.

So many outdoor swimmers are early risers, but my conditions conspire to make mornings difficult for me, especially for the complex relay of energies and focus outdoor swimming requires. If I see dawn, it's because I've been too unwell to sleep. So in summer, I become an evening swimmer instead. I swim when visitors are having their dinner, putting children to bed, going to the pub. I swim in the wake of their active days.

I swim whenever and wherever I can, delighting in the ease the warmth brings. Everywhere I go, I go with a swimming costume and towel thrown in, just in case. Any July day might become a swimming day. A fine July day without a swim is surely a mistake.

I meet friends after work at different lakes, different rivers. We seek suggestions, plot routes on maps. Revisit places we eyed up in winter or years past. We take picnics for tea, the non-swimmers amongst us happy to loiter on the shore. The swimmers swim up and down calm stretches of river, rotating onto our backs like contented otters, and loll in recesses carved out of the stone by centuries of stormier days. We linger chatting until long after the sun has gone, until the midges nipping at our hairlines become unbearable. We are determined to wring every drop of shared joy out of summer.

In July as any time, a few days of serious Lakeland rain can overwhelm a river, make it unswimmable. I've driven out west and found a mass of churning brown rapids where I expected a bridge, paths running with as much water as rivers. Days when a short walk soaks you to the skin and you look like you've been swimming through the air.

But if the air and water are warm to begin with, a rain shower on the lake is a different prospect. I've out-swum a July heatwave, chasing it across the lake as it retreats and the cloud rolls in. From the centre of the lake, I've watched my bag on the shore dry and secure as I'm lost in a galaxy of raindrops so heavy they hit the water and rise back out of it, floating globes hovering above the pocked surface. I've watched my towel on the shore soaked by a sudden squall as I've swum with the sun on my face. And just once found myself swimming through a spell, as a fine rain turned into clouds of fireflies over the water, the sun a gold lamp in the belly of each drop.

Swimming is continuous. Only the rivers are intermittent.

—Elizabeth-Jane Burnett, *Swims*

August

brambles – dog roses – squirrels gathering hazelnuts

August in the Lakes is famous for two things: tourists, and rain. Both of which William Wordsworth was already complaining about in the early 1800s. In his *Guide to the Lakes*, he recommends against visiting in August, that 'time of vacation and leisure' during which most 'strangers' take their trips. They are greeted with 'deluges of rain', rain 'settling in [...] with a vigour, and continuing with a perseverance'. Many things may have changed in the last two hundred years, but that much hasn't.

Still, it was in August when I first swam here in the lakes. A glorious bright day during my first summer living here, the end of the first year of my doctoral studies. I had moved to Grasmere in June, to an attic room in one of the many houses around Dove Cottage owned by the Wordsworth museum, all stuffed full at that time with museum workers, volunteer staff, and visiting poets and artists. Those long midsummer days were filled with learning the ways of the museum and of Grasmere, with poetry, fell-walking, elaborately themed house parties and evening picnics by the lake. But none of my new friends were swimmers, and for all those days and evenings we spent by the water, no one got in it.

On the 24th of August, I woke to a day so glorious – all hot sun and pure blue sky – that when I finished my museum work at lunchtime, I took my research outdoors, carrying my reading up to Easedale Tarn. The fells were the bright and constant green Wordsworth complained of in August, the water the same perfect blue as the sky, shimmering with sun when the breeze hit the surface.

I must have been planning to swim, because in the photos I took afterwards, I can see I had a swimming costume on under my shirt. I must have heard by then that Easedale Tarn was good for swimming. I don't remember the planning, but I remember the swim. I remember the cold of the tarn, and how surprising it was against the heat of the day. I remember standing for a long time with the water up to my thighs, wondering if it was foolish to swim alone like this, in a place I did not know. Wanting to be in the water so much, rippling with uncertainty. It was a little after three, and there was not a single other person at the tarn when I arrived. I had walked around the perimeter until I found somewhere that looked good to enter. I remember how the water – so blue from outside it – was a rich peaty brown when you were in it. How it changed the colour of my skin. How the sun collaborated with the water and my own movements, so my limbs were one moment white and glowing beneath me like stone, the next striped like fish. I could see fronds of plant life waving in the depths, a drowned forest I was flying over. It felt so good to be floating after so long trying to keep pace with natural walkers. I swam in cautious triumph, ecstatic and a little anxious. I was very aware of my aloneness, and my inexperience. I became aware of my skin, suddenly not cold anymore, but warm and warming. I swam for the stony shore, exited into warm air.

I had swum in lakes and rivers before, but not in this country, where all my outdoor swimming had been in the sea, or outdoor pools or lidos. It had taken me two months to realise that I could swim here in my new home as I'd swum in lakes in Switzerland and Canada, or rivers in France and Spain. I was already in love with Grasmere – I had been since the first night I spent here, the previous summer – but realising a life here could involve swimming in freshwater whenever I liked, that was a different offer.

That swim – the blue and green – the miniature forest – arms as fish – sun on the fells – became a kind of talisman, a moment I could return to, would find myself falling back into anytime I swam, wherever

I was. The quiet thrill of it. The sense of learning the place differently, better, more completely. How peaceful it was at the tarn, compared to the village. How all the time I was in the water, I was the only human there, only my human thoughts echoing around the crags, relieved from the psychic noise of others.

That's how it was then. A bright, hot day in August, and a whole tarn to myself.

Now, August swimming for me is an exercise in trying to balance making the most of the fleeting summer whilst avoiding holiday crowds. Evening lake swimming – amongst other locals grabbing their moments to unwind after work – and seeking those out-of-the-way spots.

Along with all the visitors come visiting friends, as during any holiday. Their plans lead me to places I would not necessarily choose myself at that busy time – a swim in Ullswater with the steamer huffing past, a swim in Coniston with red-sailed dinghies in the background, sunset swims in Rydal Water with swallows doing circuits overhead. In the water, I breathe out frustration and pretend I am on holiday too.

Sometimes these missions meld into one, as in August 2022, when meeting a friend for swim as she finished work for the day in South Cumbria led me to my first visit to High Dam.

High Dam is a man-made tarn, a piece of Cumbrian industrial heritage that had become a beloved beauty spot by the early twentieth century, as is the way of so much of the Lake District. High Dam was formed from Finsthwaite Tarn to provide power for the Stott Park Bobbin Mill, built in 1835. The water from High Dam turned a 32-foot water wheel, which was superseded in 1858 by a water turbine that required a second dam to be built, creating a smaller pool below High Dam, known as Low Dam.

In the height of a brief August heatwave, High Dam was noisy with groups with barbecues and paddleboards, families with picnics and inflatable dinghies. It is a twenty-minute walk uphill through woods to the dam from the little car park. By the time we got there in the late afternoon, some groups were walking back down carrying tired toddlers and empty coolers, but others, like us, were still arriving, or settled in for a relaxed evening in the sun. We walked more than halfway along the tarn before we found a free spot on the shore.

High Dam's ten acres are surrounded by woodland – a mix of Scots pine and larch, and coppiced birch, oak and sycamore that would have provided the wood for the bobbins at Stott Park as well as other woodland industries like charcoal burning.

The dam is a stone wall that the path around the tarn passes over. A clutch of rosebay willowherb sprouted from it, the only pink amongst the green and brown of the trees and the dry red-brown earth in August. There are wooded islands in the tarn, and even on that busy day, a heron quietly stalking the reedy channel between them. At the far end of the tarn, near where we had settled ourselves, white water lilies glowed in the sun.

In the heat that day, it felt like somewhere else to me, not Cumbria, but Canada, or Northern Europe. I've never been to Berlin, but I thought of the lakes of Berlin as I pictured them when I read Jessica J. Lee's swimming memoir. I thought of Frontenac National Park in Ontario, where I had swum a few years before with my friend Jude. It was partly the heat itself – sudden and surprising after a cold start to summer – but also the shapes of the shore, somehow, the shapes of the trees. The way the trees grew right down to the edge of the water, their roots making dusty platforms scattered with pine needles. The way the people were scattered amongst them. It felt a little unreal, as though we were in a painting or a film set.

The water was cool and strangely reddish-orange. We swam to the wall and back via the islands, leisurely amongst other swimmers, then floated amidst the lilies until we started to feel cold. I couldn't shake the feeling we'd travelled somewhere else entirely, even as I drove home on the familiar back roads, dodging flocks of pheasants in the low evening sun.

Pick your times and places, and even in hot weather, even now, you might get a quiet August swim. If you're willing to travel to more out-of-the-way spots, or swim at odd times. If you want a sunny lake in August, it will be a busy lake. But if you slip out while everyone else is having dinner, you might be blessed with a quiet dip in a solitary pool in a shady beck.

A week of Wordsworthian rain in August cools the water, heralds autumn. Red squirrels harvest the hazel trees across the road from our house, filling their larders for the winter ahead. In the cold summer of 2024, I noticed more than ever before how the nights lengthen as the month progresses. By mid-month, I felt the dark half of the year arriving with bats and blankets, twilight at 9pm.

By the end of the month, it is 7pm when the sun drops down behind the fells, throws my favourite little beach into early shadow. Autumn is on the wind.

Water remembers: all the stages of your life, the lives that have come before and the mountains it has fallen on that no longer exist.

—Bethany Handley, *My Body is a Meadow*

September

turning leaves – acorns – rowan berries ripening

One moment, it is high summer, the woods around the lake lush green, the water warm and silky, sparkling with sun, each parcel of beach claimed and covered in people – then it rains, for a day, or a week – and when the rain stops, the people have gone, the colours have changed, the air tastes different.

You walk to the lake after 5pm and there are no groups there with their picnics and paddleboards, only one young woman quietly reading, and a couple walking a dog on the far shore. The lake is still warm where the sun touches it, but cold beneath. A few brown leaves turn on the still surface, early adopters of coming fall. The trees on the shore are darkening out of their summer green, a kind of tarnished bronze, green-brown in the dark mirror of the water. The sun is already dropping behind the western fells as you swim, and you stretch into it, swimming up the lake parallel to the eastern shore to keep your face in it for as long as you can. That evening, you will see a red deer grazing in the small meadow in the village centre, a visitor from winter, and a yellow harvest moon will rise over the rooftops, not quite full. Owls call out their new territories from the trees, the most you have heard of them for months. There is no mistaking it, then: summer has slipped away while your back was turned.

How does it come as a surprise every year? This shift into autumn? The suddenness of the change? You close your eyes on a summer afternoon for just a breath, and when you open them again all the leaves have fallen, the woods are in shadow, and when you release it, your breath hangs like the mist in the hollows. Each day seems to shorten half an hour at a time. You begin the month trying to hold on to the light. By the equinox, you have begun to adjust to the dark. You light candles and the fire in the evenings.

Some Septembers bring a shimmer of late heat, just when you have given it over: a stolen summer with shrinking days. Some Septembers bring weeks of rain that wash all residual warmth from the water and fill the rivers to overflowing. How you swim in September depends on what variety of September arrives at the closing down of the summer.

A swim on a fine day in September with sun warming the still surface of a lake is an entirely different proposal to a swim on a stormy autumn day with rain and hail pelting you as you try to change, fingers and toes numb as though in midwinter. Picking your body of water and window of weather is a particular skill. If it has been a hot summer, it is easy to forget how quickly the temperature of both the air and your body can drop once the weather turns or the sun goes down. A September heatwave can trick you into thinking it is still summer, but when the sun drops, there is a bitter chill like a coming frost in it, mist swirling around the ankles of the trees. The air smells of leaf mould, fungi, a hint of woodsmoke. Something deep and rich like oakmoss.

September 2024 brought a surprise heatwave – the finest weather all year – still, golden days and mild starlit nights to make up for a summer that never arrived. A warm, bright day at this time of year always feels like a gift, but that year in particular, when a Saturday in mid-July gave rain-soaked highs of only 11°C, it seemed especially precious. For one week, it was the autumn swimming weather of my dreams: the kind I held in mind each time I gazed into the heaving white and brown of a river too wild to swim in after rain, or a balmy river pool cluttered with summer holiday people and all the rubbish they left behind. So many years and so many rivers and tarns I had wistfully imagined on a bright September day: the water still warm, or warmish, the people gone. Sun on rowan berries and turning leaves. The perfect balance.

It had felt like autumn all the way through the cold, damp August. Mushrooms in the woods, the trees already turning. When the late heat arrived out of gloom on the 16th, I chased the sun to the lake in the afternoon, almost missing it as I'd missed the shift in daylight hours under all the cloud. It was the first time I'd been in the lake in weeks, between work taking me away from home, and wild rain and blustery storms on my return. It felt like summer was rising and setting at the same time. Strange season, where the start meets the end. There was one other human swimming that evening – two humans alongside all the nonhuman life and leaves in the golden light. It felt like the very archetype of an autumn swim.

The next day, I didn't believe the heat would stay, and almost missed it again, tracking the falling sun up to High Dam when I realised my error in the afternoon. When we reached the tarn, the sun was already balanced on the very tips of the tall pines on the opposite shore. For every item of clothing I shed, it stepped one more pace away from us, retreating over the darkening water. One of the things I'd remembered most of all from my summer swim two years earlier at High Dam was the redness of the water – peat or iron, I wasn't sure – but I stepped in with my face lit orange above the water and my limbs orange below it, the water a dark veil between the two. Half the tarn was in shadow by the time I launched myself forward, the sun splitting into glowing amber skeins between the trees, and the whole scene looking increasingly like a Group of Seven painting. The dam and the trees around it were in rich sun still, and I swam towards them in a fantasia of autumn colour, weaving the ambers and reds of the blazing reflections into the dark water between.

A group of swimmers had arrived a few minutes after us and were shivering and yelping as they got in, as I floated by the dam in the glorious glow, knowing I would have to swim back into the shadow.

The sun was gone entirely and the tarn in rapidly cooling twilight by the time I clambered back out, dripping, my breath rising out of me like the ghost of summer. As I fumbled into my clothes, a huge peachy harvest moon rose over the trees.

We walked back down into a different season. On the drive home, the fields moved with a tide of mist, lit in improbable pastels by the last glimmer of sunset, deer floating through it like ships.

On the 18th and 19th, I manage to make it to the lake in full daylight, early in the afternoon, and am met with two lake swims equally splendid in gold and blue, the heron quietly stalking around in the background. More copper leaves sailing alongside me each day.

The heat lingers longer than I could have hoped. On the 20th, I have time to head to one of my favourite river swimming spots in Borrowdale. The water here is luminous whatever the weather, channelled through the volcanic rock into a series of deep gorges and small falls. But in this September sun, filtered through turning leaves on the oaks on the shore, and again by the fallen leaves traveling downstream, it is like a vision.

I enter the river in the shadow of its stone walls. The sun is sitting low just over the little waterfall that marks the upper end of this narrow channel, the spray turning to gold as it rises towards the blue sky. Everything is glinting and sparkling as I swim upstream towards it. When I reach the point the light reaches the water, my face ignites, droplets on my eyelashes casting rainbows. It is like swimming into light, not water. I dive in and out of it. I feel like a fish, shining as a scaled thing. I don't want to get out.

Grasmere the evening before the equinox is resplendent in gold. Only a lone brown leaf turning on the mirrored surface, and the moth I scoop out and carry back to shore – an Autumnal Rustic – remind me it is September and not July. The mirror begins to mist over as the fells swallow the sun.

On the rocks along the shore that get the last drop of noon sun at winter solstice, there is a grey wagtail bobbing, drawing the gold light into its sun-yellow belly as though to say, *You know where to find it now, when you need it. Which you will.*

The next day, the weather turns. I have one more river swim, out west, in a favourite spot in the Esk where I never seem to catch the light. Missing the light often means having the river to myself though, which is a great compensation. I turn and turn in the dark water like the leaves carried downstream. It is beautiful, but it is definitely autumn. No more pretending it could still be summer.

September 2025 begins wet, and chilly, an entirely different being. By mid-month, the shallow fringe of the lake is thick with fallen leaves and fat acorns, swollen with water, which you must wade through to enter. I know it won't be long until it is too cold for me to walk in with bare feet, and I am trying to enjoy it whilst I can, though I don't like to not be able to see where I am stepping clearly. The leaves tickle my toes and ankles. I hope there are no bottle tops or fishing hooks hiding amongst them. I get out of the water when the sun goes. It is 6pm, and across the lake a tawny owl clears its throat, lets out a first mournful *hooo hoooooooooo.*

The month blazes out with a week of glorious sunshine, but this year, it comes with frosts in the mornings. Days that rise from freezing at dawn to sunburn in the afternoon, and back to freezing. The sun in the day isn't enough to make up for the cold at night, and the water temperature drops and drops. By the fifth day of it, my finger joints are seizing up as I swim.

October comes in on a storm, and the next time I swim, it will be glove season.

September

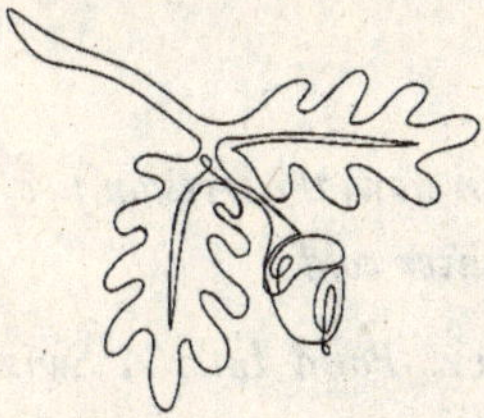

Real autumn now, the trees on fire, leaves blowing wildly, the water cold.

—Al Alvarez, *Pond Life: A Swimmer's Journal*

October

mushrooms – sweet chestnuts – redwings

October is peak autumn in the Lakes: the bracken on the fells chestnut brown, and the trees resplendent in their turning, a spectrum from green to yellow through orange and all the reds. When you walk or swim beneath them, the leaves are like stained glass against the sky, and they throw their colours onto every body of water near them: lake, tarn, river, puddle. Everything reflects autumn's rusted rainbow. On bright days, it shines amber, gold, copper – the sun igniting the sweetened leaves into echoes of flame. On misty days when the fell tops are swallowed by cloud or seem to steam in the rain, the palette is darker and richer. Burgundy, ochre.

Then under and in and on the trees, all the colours of fungi mushrooming up. The unlikely purple of amethyst deceivers, snowflakes on red riding hood of fly agaric, stratified sand of turkey tails. Toadstools the exact same burnt umber as beech leaves, sprouting all along fallen beech trees. The ghostly white umbrellas of porcelain mushrooms growing high up on a branch.

When the porcelain mushrooms return, so do the winter thrushes. Huge flocks of redwings settling on the common. The woods are busy with red squirrels moving their hoards. The horse chestnut throws down conkers that shine in the rain like polished furniture. If you can catch it at just the right time, a sweet chestnut offers delicious bounty. Some years I fill my pockets and bag with nuts to roast on the fire, some years all I get is empty shells underfoot. That's October. Storms or splendour, and everything shining and glistening either way. I used to think of autumn as a kind of dying, now I understand it as a different kind of growth. A shedding of what no longer serves us, a recentring of energy in our core.

October swimming is a long drawn-out argument with the growing cold. A few chilly days and frosty nights and the lake temperature drops decisively, will not get enough sun to rise again till spring. A soft mild spell can follow an October cold snap, but the warmer air won't do much to alter the cooling of the water. Each drop of sun is to be savoured now, each moment of warmth to be gathered up and swaddled around you against the coming winter.

I like to see how long I can keep swimming with bare feet and hands before I have to give in to wearing insulated socks and gloves. Each swim without them might be the last of the year. You never know the last one when you're in it, only afterwards, when you can't repeat it. My swims get shorter as the lake gets colder, until my finger joints and toes can't take it anymore, until the pain the cold brings is immediate and interrupting.

I would love to be able to keep swimming all year without the thermal insulation of socks and gloves, but for the years I have swum all winter, they are what enable it for me. For that, I am thankful, even if I hate the way they remove me from the water, the way they alter my sense of my body in space, of how I extend into the water. The cold, wet weight of them to be carried home. How impossible it is to dry them out well in the cave of our house.

The gloves come first, but both later than they used to.

I used to think my inability to regulate my body temperature – the faulty internal thermostat I experience as part of a general dysfunction of my autonomic nervous system – would mean I would never develop any cold tolerance.

But year by year, little by little, my body has got better at adjusting to the cold. It might be a tiny, crawling shift, but it is a shift. In parallel, I have learnt my body's limits, and how to adjust for them.

I am still a cold person, with cold person problems, but I know what kinds of external cold I can cope with, what kinds I can't. I better know how to warm myself up, and how to be cold safely. I know how to listen to my body, and what it can or cannot tolerate on any given day.

Every October, I have to relearn this. Remind myself I can get in the water, that I can tolerate more than I once would have imagined. That I can flourish in autumn, just in a different way.

The lake in October is a receptacle for fallen leaves. They swim with you in the absence of other humans. Sometimes there are people fishing along the shore. Who gets a spot in the lingering light is a matter of timing, and luck. On a gentle sunny day, the lake light is golden, so rich you can almost taste it.

But a cold wind in October can shift the season, can shift my pain levels from drizzly to stormy. I always forget a little quite how hard the change in seasons hits me. October always seems to bring a flare along with the cold and the falling leaves.

We stock up on sunflower hearts and fill the bird feeder, bringing constant traffic to the front window – blue tits and great tits and flocks of long-tailed tits, the odd nuthatch and noisy finches, spilling over from the back garden. If we let the feeder empty, the birds hop along the windowsill, glare in at us, tap on the glass with their beaks.

Before the end of the month, the clocks change, and an hour of afternoon light is lost. It gets harder and harder to get myself out when there will still be light on the water. I miss it once, twice, chasing it back along the shore. Short, chilly swims, and the fire lit at home after. And that's how I meet Halloween, looking the dark in the face, trying not to be afraid of it, and what it will bring.

At the sharp edge of sensation, the cut of the ice, or in the silk of the warming lake, like moments before sleep, the lake is a threshold. Memories swell. Sensation floats at the surface like fog.

—Jessica J Lee, *Turning*

November

tawny owls courting – dippers singing – frost

November can be hard. The days seem suddenly terribly short, and so often grey and lightless, relentlessly cold, nothing much to cheer them.

But a bright day in November is truly spectacular. If the trees have kept their leaves through October, they are at their richest and most colourful now. All amber and copper and long shadows, and the low light thick and sweet as honey when it flows. The trees that hang onto their leaves seem all the brighter for their bare neighbours. The lake multiplies them, amplifies their bright noise.

By the end of the month, the yellows of early autumn are gone. What remains is the auburn of foxes and red squirrels. Rusty beech leaves that will linger through winter, bringing brightness to the monochrome world of the wood. Even in the lowest of November light, the beech leaves seem to glow with all that stored energy, luminous orange in the gloom.

On a grey day, the colours of the trees in the lake are glorious. The bright orange of the beeches and sycamores, greens of the firs. The birches mostly bare now, purple in their skin, and others hanging onto slivers of yellows and reds – all doubled and stretched by the lake.

I used to think of November as grey before I lived here, but now I think of it as burnished copper. Thin light on a rusting world.

And there is still song in it. One November day walking home from swimming, I heard a burst of beautiful song float up over the wall from the lakeshore, looked down, and there was a dipper singing to a hidden companion. It was the first dipper I'd seen since spring. During the swim itself, three grey wagtails fluttered over me in the thin rays of sun filtering through the trees as it sank behind them. No heron that day, but black-headed gulls, and a buzzard keening as it crossed the water. The next day, the dipper was singing from the same spot again, with gangs of long-tailed tits flitting overhead as I changed, annoying the wren who was sheltering in mossy trees. There were goldcrests and blue tits singing, and a grey wagtail who landed next to me, nodded, then took off.

November brings the first real ice. Frosted leaves that don't thaw in the shadow. By later in the month, they are trapped under contours of ice in puddles and the tarns and maybe even the hem of the lake. A clear day means a cold night, which means frost in the mornings, an inversion filling the valley with mist that lingers over the water when the sun finally inches over the fells. There may be snow on the tops of the fells, maybe even a first snowfall in the village. And all of this reflected in the polished surface of the lake.

That's my ideal November swim, when the water is smooth as glass, the heron is doing rounds, and there's enough sun to sit drying in your towel in the dregs of it.

On other days, the heron hunches into itself against the icy wind, and I do too. Those are the days it feels most back-endish, not so much autumn as a long dark passage into winter. An icy wind driving onto the shore reminds me that even if you go out in your swimming gear very much intending to swim, you don't have to get in. No one gets to decide but you. Sometimes it is warmer in the water than out of it in the wind. Some days you stand so long with your feet in the waves and the sun on the back of your knees you think you can't go any further, but you do, you can, reminding yourself that in a month, it will be starting to get lighter again. Sometimes it is worth it to get in, sometimes it is not. Your body is the only one who knows.

Swimming all year is also learning to listen to your body when it tells you to just watch the heron from the shore for a while, and head home for a hot bath instead.

At twilight, all the trees seem to echo with owl calls, a relay from one end of the valley to the other. I hear couples cooing to each other in the special voices they use for courting, and know that spring will bring owlets.

On a cold day at the end of the month, I meet a red stag on the edge of the common. The antler report he gives me says, *Come down from the high ground, winter is almost here. Stay close to the trees and we will be all bare branches amongst bare branches, all winter branches together.*

My swims are shorter now, even on a calm and sunny day. Breath pooling out from my warm body in the cold water and mingling with the lingering mist.

Except, if I time it right, and the weather allows, there is surprising warmth in the sun. Even in the cold water, the sun reflecting on my face is warm through the cold air, and the sun reflecting off the mirror of the water back onto my face is even warmer. Swimming lets me feel it, even in these short and darkening days. It lets me feel it and gets me out in it. It encourages me to open myself to this small sliver of light.

Before I swam all winter, I would never have thought to sit out in it like I do now, especially not wearing only a towel, letting the sun touch as much of my skin as I can.

By this time of year, I am seeking apricity when I swim – the warmth of the sun even when the air is cold. I hold onto it like a float in the grey gloom. I am using it to keep my head above water.

Each lake is a page
we have not written on.
The mist is breath

suspended. Stars shiver.
There's a ghost
of a winter moon.

It is late December:
[…]
The cold is a hurt
we return to, over and over.

—Clare Shaw, *Night Swimming, Derwentwater*

December

frozen holly berries – waxwings – geminids

In the short days of midwinter, it is too easy for me to miss the light entirely. I get distracted working, or wait to see if the cloud lifts, or a hint of sun in the distance touches the village. Grasmere is a small bowl of a valley, a cupped palm, as I put it once. In midwinter, the sun barely reaches in at all, spends an hour or two before noon creeping down the fells and trees and houses, a couple of hours after creeping back up. Mountain twilight begins around 2pm, long before civil twilight.

Meeting daylight on its inward or outwards journey becomes increasingly unlikely if your body is not amenable to movement in the morning. If I have anything much at all to do other than to try and meet daylight, it becomes near impossible to get out of the house in the short window when the sun is high enough to peer over the lip of the valley's bowl.

I think of those communities in steep mountain valleys in the Italian alps and Norway that use vast mirrors to reflect light into their villages in winter, like the Egyptians used to light the tunnels in a pyramid. I fantasise more than ever of owning a home on the east side of the valley, high enough up to keep the light, with big windows to let it in, looking out over the shaded woods on the west. I glare at the sunlit windows of second homes with dull, aching envy.

So often I go just a little too late, reach the lake with the watery sun already falling away behind the fells, or a shroud of cloud lying over them. There is a heavy greyness on a day like that, all the colours muted. The water greyish-brown like the fells, like the woods. The vivid colours of November swept away by a bitter wind.

But even on a cold, dank day like that, even when I miss the light, there is something to find at the lake. A meeting of the ice in the core of my bones with the near-ice of the water. Something like original response.

My swims now are brief. The cold begins to cut through my socks and gloves, and it is harder to both get in, and to get out and changed. When the cold water hits my chest, I count strokes and concentrate on my breathing until I begin to relax a little.

If I manage to catch the light, I might be lucky enough to see the lake's ghost rising from its body as mist and grey wagtail. I find the heron occupying my usual swim spot whilst I seek the sun further along the shore.

On the way home, lit windows glow like beacons in the dusk. So often at this time of year, it seems to get lighter at dusk, not darker. In the strange light-dark, every lit building looks like the empire of light, quite painterly and implausible.

A fiery sunset reminds me that even a December twilight has more lumens to offer than the cave house in winter. And colour, at least, wild and vivid colour.

The weather fluctuates between rain and ice, snow and sun. The window of any given day I can and want to swim in gets smaller and smaller.

Most years friends join me for a solstice swim, either on the day itself or as close as weather and commitments will allow, a tradition that began the first winter I swam through. That year, when a swim on a grey day in December was a new triumph, our post-solstice swim brought the loss of my first, new and expensive waterproof camera. I felt it fall away from me almost as soon as my feet left the ground and I moved to swim out into the lake. We tried to dive for it, but in our buoyant winter wetsuits, we stood no chance against the cold water. I searched for the camera once spring came, and have tried, increasingly aimlessly and hopelessly, every year since, but I have to accept it now as belonging to the lake, not me. Sometimes I imagine it rising back up without me one day, like Excalibur held aloft by the lady of the lake.

There was a dead pike on the shore that day, the only time I've ever seen one up close. When I was a child, pike terrified me, thanks largely to the scene in *The Sword in the Stone* when Wart, as a minnow, is chased by one. Its huge snapping, overlocking teeth. The last photo I took on the drowned camera was of the dead pike, thinking of it as a kind of rehabilitation.

I used to tell people there was a great pike at the bottom of Grasmere, the monster of the lake, a story I'm sure I borrowed from a friend who first used it to tease me. As I did in childhood, I took the fear and shared it, made it into a joke to pass on. I thought maybe the pike on the shore that day was the great pike, not so great after all. The camera is down there with the pike now. It belongs to them.

I want to sleep through December but I forget how to sleep at the right times. It's dark for so long so much of the time, I lose the boundaries of day and night. I am wide awake at 4am, useless at noon.

I try to make sure I go out in the daylight, whatever the weather. I take vitamin D. I prioritise daylight over work, daylight over anything.

When the sun does shine, it is dazzling. It turns everything along the lake shore a pale gold in its glare – reeds, trees, walls.

Through the years, I have found the spots I can reach along the shore to swim from that keep the light the longest. There is a beach I call the winter beach because it holds the sun for a good hour even at solstice. That is the clock of lake. If Grasmere were a henge, or a passage burial, that spot would be the altar, the mouth of the tomb.

It is there I go on a bright December day, knowing I can swim out and back and dry and change held by the thin gold light. That I can be glazed in its glitter too.

Sometimes there is ice in the shallows that I crack cautiously to step over to enter the lake. Sometimes there is snow on the beach.

I go down in my snow boots with grips on. I go with my warmest clothes to layer up.

Each time I go to the winter beach, it reminds me that the winter world is not asleep at all. The birds are as busy as ever. I watch them as I swim, and as I change they move around me. Shoals of long-tailed tits swoop from tree to tree, trilling. Noisy blue tits and great tits hop from bush to bush. A wren shouts from the sidelines. There is a robin carolling from the mossy oak, goldcrests cheeping. I love to be in their company, they who never expect me to explain anything to them, yet always have something to say to me. Best of all, I love the grey wagtails, who always remind me that light is still here, even in the darkest times, even if hidden under an outstretched wing of grey. Under it, there is sun, and the best way to see it is reflected in the water.

December

I think about loving swimming the way you love somebody. How a kiss happens, gravitational.

—Leanne Shapton, *Swimming Studies*

January

hoar frost – starlight – new antlers

January has its two faces, like the god it is named for, himself named for a doorway or passage, open to both or all directions. A month of endings and beginnings, of transition and travel. There are days when it feels like the sun never rises at all, and all hours blend in to one long purplish twilight; days when the winter sun is so bright for its short outing it feels like a visitation from another realm. Dry bright days when everything is white with hoar frost, shimmering in the light, like a fantasy of winter. The fells white as they stretch down to the lake, white mist on the still water cut through with sun. Everything the sun touches glittering. A palette of blue, white and gold. Wavy ice like old glass at the edge of the water that cracks beneath my feet as I step on it, tentatively, my feet encased in thick neoprene.

These days, I almost love winter. These days, I remember why I swim all through it.

When it's bright and still like this, I don't wear my full wetsuit anymore. I've realised over the years which parts of my body I can bear to get cold, and which I can't. Most of the winter now I will swim in a neoprene top over a long-sleeved swimming costume to protect my neck and shoulders, 5mm socks and gloves, and if there is any wind at all, a hat.

I step into the lake, and the water goes over my socks, hits my bare legs. I keep moving forward until I am standing waist-deep. When my legs are numb, I am ready to glide forward. I breathe out as I make an arrow of my body, in as I return my arms to my sides. It is never easy, to put my chest and shoulders under, but habit makes it less hard. I know the reward I get for it, to be in the lake, to have that shining mist at eye level, to be part of the landscape, not an observer of it. I count breaths, count strokes. Turn back before I think I need to. Turn my face to the light. Make sure I get out with the sun still clear above the fells from the winter beach.

When I get out, I take off my cold wet things as quickly as possible, hang them over the mossy oak to drip. I dry my feet and put my thick wool socks on, but I don't get dressed, not yet. I put myself in the sun wrapped up in my towel.

Most days, a grey wagtail joins me as I bask, that little reminder. They seem to love the sun as much as I do.

One thing I've finally learnt after over four decades of living with chronic illness is that it's far more important to attend to the weather – inside and outside the body – than the calendar.

In January more than any other time of year, I follow this. I want to begin the year as I need it to continue. I save my new year swim for a fine day, not necessarily the first. If the sun comes on the second instead, then that is the time to swim.

I will swim the new year in at my own pace, on my own terms. I will swim it in with the sun on my face and an afternoon moon rising over snowy fells, the sun white as the moon in the frozen cloud.

I prefer always a cold, clear day to a milder, damp one. Let the mud turn to ice, and let everything be thick with frost. Frost so thick it is like fur on everything, even the sun. The whole world white and shining.

In the first decade I lived here, the lake froze over entirely some winters. It froze then froze again, the ice white with snow or frost, dark patterns drawn on it by the movement of the water below. They always looked to me like diagrams of nerve cells I learnt to drawn at school. It hasn't frozen like that in the years I've been winter swimming, or not for more than a few hours. One year, it froze overnight then broke up the next day in a wild driving wind, which blew all the breaking up sheets of ice towards the shore like smashed window panes. We did not get too close that day, and I certainly didn't swim.

Even more than in December, in January I try and save the short hours I am active in daylight to spend in the daylight. I swim, or I walk on the common. Sometimes I manage to do both. A swim amongst birds then a walk amongst deer, noting the progression of the season in the progression of their antlers. By mid-month, I find them swaddled in velvet and already three-pronged. There are flocks of redwing and long-tailed tits. Ravens and buzzards moving around high above me. I see hunting owls, attentive robins, startled woodcocks.

A sudden mild day in January can feel like a mini-spring, all the birds singing through unpredicted glimpses of sun, milder air, and everything defrosting and dripping with snowmelt.

Already these few weeks' travel from the solstice means the sun peeks over Loughrigg to reach the lakeshore again by noon – about twenty minutes earlier than at New Year. It will stay on the winter beach for a delicious hour, when it barely touches our house at all. I swim now entirely as a light-seeking exercise. It has been so long since summer I can't imagine it anymore, but I know this thin yellow winter light on the water is possible. I know I can sit in it for an hour and the world will feel more tolerable. I can watch the mist move over it and the water move and still in the wind.

By the third week of the month, the light is lingering noticeably longer. On the winter beach, it stays until 2pm, a very luxurious window of light, suddenly. I begin to relax a little, the panic to catch it simmering down.

Down at my favourite spot, which I have surrendered to the solstice, the light is touching the shore at midday again. One extraordinarily bright freezing beautiful day, a friend joins me for a lunchtime swim and we find a heron waiting for us down there. We all seem as dazzled by the light as each other, and it lets us watch it for a good ten minutes before it lifts off and away from scrutiny. There is snow on the tops, and the lake is so still and so clear it feels like you should be able to see the Milky Way in it in the middle of the day.

The sun is still just stretching out towards the little beach at 1.40pm.

By the end of the month, it will be 2pm. The first few snowdrops have pushed up through the muddy ice of the churchyard, the first new green of the year. There is still so much more winter to get through, but there is new growth under the surface. I have to remember this in the storms of February. It is there, no matter how bleak and hopeless it looks from above.

All winter the river was one creature.
It shrank and expanded, but maintained
its borders. I saw to the bottom. Firm sinew.

Clear curve. I swam in it long as I could bear.

—Emily Hasler, *Difference*

February

snowdrops – catkins – crocuses

February used to bring the deepest snows of winter. Now more often it is a month of wild rainstorms, the kind that make swimming impossible, or reckless. If not high winds, the kind of set-in foggy mizzle that erases the fells and the lake inch by inch.

But even on a grey day at the start of the month, you can see the light coming back. There is light at 5pm, even if the light has been half-light all day. I take comfort in the old tales. If the weather is bad on the 1st, the Cailleach can't gather her firewood, and will call the spring in sooner.

I used to find February the hardest month, so far from light in either direction. But the more I've paid attention, the more I've found the colour in it all the same.

The woods can seem so drab in February, so incredibly sparse. If there is sun, the sun is watery and pale. But from within the lake, the sun on the bare trees makes their grey bark glow with a metallic sheen. If the sky is blue, the lake is blue. Blue sky, blue lake, shining trees and blonde reeds between them. Sometimes enough sun through the remnants of rain to make a rainbow over the fells. The wind cold enough to make your teeth hurt when you smile, all the small birds tweeting and a heron flyover.

Sometimes no sun at all but also no wind, no rain, and a swim through grey into grey, like swimming off the end of the known world, the fells erased in mist and low cloud. A heron on rocks and bare trees reflected in the still grey water, but nothing beyond them.

Sometimes the cloud hugging the high fells, and the lake overcast but calm. The colour of the fells shifting, a washed-out grey-green presaging spring.

On days like this, I may be the only swimmer in the afternoon, but the lake shore may be busy with other users, walkers, people fishing. Some winter days, there are rows of fishing rods set up all along the shore, beeping away to themselves. When there are people fishing, the herons are never far away, watching and waiting. In turn, I watch them shouting at the anglers and doing circuits over the water as I swim.

Another day, there is so much dilute sun it makes my eyes water.

The heron flies over with light caught in its wings. The little boat at the winter beach is underwater. Under the bare trees, it looks like a lost scene from *The Lady of Shalott*.

I find the neck of an old glass medicine bottle under the trees, risen out of the soil after the rain. It is pale ice-blue. I hold it up to the sun, which is sitting higher over the fells every day. I hold the sun in its blue circle. Soon enough, there will be plenty of light at the far end of the lake again.

February too often feels like a month to endure. And that is enough. To keep going is its own kind of triumph.

In 2024, between endless rain and saving energy for work, I didn't swim once in the whole of the month of February. That year, when I did get back in the water on the 3rd of March, there was blue sky and billowing clouds over snow-capped fells, a heron flyover and a pair of wagtails heralding the sun, reminding me it's better to wait till the right time, even if it means missing an entire month of the year. Swimming through does not mean always swimming. Timing is everything.

I am not sure where the shape of me ends and the dark water begins.

—Nina Mingya Powles, *Small Bodies of Water*

March

primroses – celandine – forget-me-nots

March has one foot in winter, one foot in spring. In like a lion, out like a lamb – though it's never so simple. Our lions and lambs co-exist in Grasmere – as they do on the summit of Helm Crag – the lamb always at the foot of the lion, the lion always holding the lamb in its arms.

The crocuses are joined by primroses now, neon yellow against the drab of wintry earth. In boggy corners, yellow celandines open their hands to hold the light. At the tarn, the frogs are singing – a strange, undulating mass of song. The birds are all homemaking. As I work, a goldcrest visits the window all day, gathering cobwebs to shore up its nest.

There is blossom opening. Magnolias start to spread their great archaic blooms against the sky.

There are chilly swims in biting wind and choppy water. There are still mizzly days when the birdsong vanishes into mist, black-headed gulls still in their white winter livery swooping out of it at the shore.

March 2025 brought unusually mild and bright days, and with them the first swims of the year when I could linger just a little, take a little time in the water, still gloved and booted and cold as soon as the sun dropped, but so needed. I knew the cold would come back before spring really settled in, but the respite was so welcome.

In the water, I breathe. Stretch. Fold the sky into the fells, the fells into the sun. Breathe. Float on. Keep living.

The colours of the valley are changing again. The washed-out greige of late winter joined by a first few flickers of early, uncertain green.

On the equinox, it is warmer in the sun than it had been the previous summer. Cold nights and cold water a reminder it is only March.

My swims get longer, and later. After the equinox, the sun does not dip and vanish from my little beach until 5.30pm, and I want to clap in delight.

The globe is shifting into a rhythm that syncs with mine again.

It all gets easier from here. I have to remind myself of this on the days that feel like winter, when it feels like I might never be warm again.

Every time I swim, I notice more signs of the changing season. A new leaf, a new bloom, a new bird.

I swim in the lake, mostly, at this time of year. Where I know my boundaries and its. But in March 2024, a dear friend comes to visit and we go to a favourite upland river a good month earlier than I ever have before. The water is always cold there, and I expect it to be brutal. The trees are winter bare, but the rocks green with moss. There is no sun, but no rain either, little wind. The landscape seen as a whole gives the impression of grey-green, a thin early-spring green, the colour of lichen and slate. From the rocky shore looking down, the river is a dark blue-green fissure. Wet bark. Winter sky. But the water is so clear here. In it, part of it, we find it bright turquoise against the rocky river channel, the brightest thing around.

I wear my socks and gloves and neoprene top, keep my head above water. My friend, who loves the cold as much as I dread it, swims in a bikini, dives under the surface and spins her body against the flow. It feels barely colder than some of our swims here much later in the year. As we pick up our things to walk away, the cloud parts to reveal a tiny patch of blue sky.

It opens something, a possibility, and the following year I swim there in the first mild spell again. I don't swim under the water and follow the current with the fish like I do in summer, but just to be there is glorious.

A few days after that earliest ever river swim in March 2024, I have my earliest ever gloveless and sockless lake swim. Not deliberately. My head is still in work when I am rushing to pack my swimming bag and get to the lake in the light, and I leave my socks and gloves drying in the house.

At the lake, I face the choice – swim without them, or miss the light. I survey the water, perfectly still, the way the sun seems to cut straight through it to the lake floor. So clear, so peaceful. I step in cautiously. I know my feet can take the temperature because the week before, I'd stopped for a paddle, too short on time and energy for a swim. I had taken my socks and shoes off then, rolled up my jeans, and the water, though cold, was not painful.

Now I stood in it, contemplating my choices. I had the shore to myself. The lake was so calm. The sun so inviting. The water blue with reflected sky. On the shore, the grey-greens of earlier in the month are being supplanted by something brighter. The vivid yellow of daffodils, the fresh green of new grass.

But I worried about my hands. I had been talking with my friend about how I'd noticed my cold tolerance had improved in these years of all-season swimming, even though the improvement is marginal. My hands have been the most marginal of those improvements.

I stood there, weighing it up, my feet growing slowly more comfortable with the notion. I walked in until my fingertips were touching the water, and swilled them around, letting them lead the decision.

The sun is buttery on the water, the trees. A wagtail passes by and tells me to go for it, and I do. A short, sharp swim. The cold cuts at my joints, is a knife through knuckle of my right hand, but the surface of the water is already warming, just slightly.

I'd have been more comfortable wearing gloves, but the pain is not terrible, and subsides quickly. And it is worth it, this time, the clean cut of pain for the glory of lake light and to be submerged in all that beauty.

It is the 30th of March, and I sit drying in my towel in the sun until after 5pm, my yellow toenails rhyming with the sun.

I am learning all the time. I am learning to respond to what is there in the moment, whether it is in my body, or the water. I am learning to measure my expectations and my experience more carefully against the present. I am learning all the things that can mean, all the things it can lead to. I am learning how to hunker down into the ground of myself in winter, how to weather the frost, how to come back up out in spring.

To swim is to witness metamorphosis, in our environment, in ourselves. To swim is to accept all the myriad conditions of life.

—Bonnie Tsui, *Why We Swim*

April

daffodils – dog violets – wood sorrel

The fellsides are frothing with white blackthorn blossom and hawthorn blossom.

The path through the woods is lit by tiny dog violets and the drooping porcelain cups of wood sorrel, pink-veined, turning their insides up to the sun when it shines. All the birds are nesting, busy, loud.

Under the trees and along the dry stone walls, the small red bells of bilberry flowers promising berries in the summer.

By the lake shore, a scattering of white wood anemones between the foot of the great beeches and the scrubby birches, stars in greening sky.

The trees overhanging the lake are all catkins and buds. The leaves are unfurling, one by one, then many. It is how it goes.

The fells and their reflections are putting on their spring green now, tentative and hopeful. Greener and brighter every day.

A few sunny days, and the surface of the lake begins to warm, just a little, enough to remind me that summer is possible. I am thinking of shedding layers for real now. I try it little by little. A swim without socks on a calm day when the sun suggests a later date. One day, I forget my gloves again, manage a decent swim without them without too much pain.

When I sit on the shore drying, I am joined by flotillas of ducklings, squeaking and nibbling around my toes. They squeak with every little step they take, *squeak squeak squeak.*

Sometimes a mouse runs out of the tree and sits next to me for a moment.

On the walk home, owls hunting, deer creeping around. I see a first bluebell almost opening in Banerigg, a first bluebell flower poking up on its stalk in Ladywood – though all around them only leaves as far as my eye could search. I see a first few wood sorrel flowers closing against the dipped sun at 6pm. There are raindrops on new buds and celandines, and songbirds everywhere. One roe deer surprised to see a sole human wandering through her trees.

The blossom comes out on our little apple tree. One day, I spot a moulting roe deer doing her best work on a holiday home garden, eating all the sweet flowers. I see the first Welsh poppy of the spring in bright sun yellow, tiny puddles of sleeping lambs.

By the second week of April, I might have my first swim of the year that could be called an evening swim. You can get in the water at 6pm, swim in the light, and find it still beautifully sunny by the time you get out to get dried, the sun just dropping behind the fells at 7pm. If you're lucky, a grey wagtail will be sitting in a tree above you as you change, pick up your stuff, head home.

The first light and warm days of spring are always such a relief to me.

If the weather is fine, there may come a day when if you squint away the patchy leaf-cover, you could think it summer, that you have made it already.

In mid-month, I look up and see one swallow flying over, then another close on its tail. I hear an owl clearing its throat, but no sign of any owlets yet.

The dominant sound of the woods is *chiff chaff chiff chaff chiff chaff.*

One buck has shed his velvet already, another has kept his, a reminder we all have our own measures of time, our own internal clocks.

Yellow flag irises are bursting up amongst the daffodils and around the tarn. Bracken is uncurling its spiralled fiddleheads.

At the end of the month, I see my first butterfly, a peacock opening its wings to the sun.

April can have its sudden snows, its sudden freezes. April can have its storms and its winds. The gloves and socks and hat go back on. You think you might never be warm again. But even with snow, you know where it is heading.

You grit your teeth now and swim on, because it is really spring. Soon you will be back at the start.

April

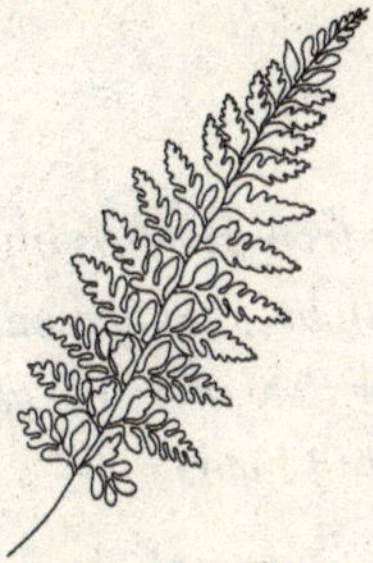

The river emerges from greyness into deep green colour and clear light. […] Spreading my arms wide, I let the slow flow carry me gently along through shadow and light.

—Rose Macaulay, *Personal Pleasures*

May (again)

damselflies – mayflies – tormentil

May, again. Maybe it starts with snow, maybe sun. Either way, there are daffodils bobbing in the wind by the lake shore. The first bluebells open or opening. Soon, the woods and fellsides will be covered with them.

Little leaves unfurl. The valley greens day by day.

One day, the columbines suddenly appear, open-winged, in front of the house, then the first rose.

There are woodpeckers calling to each other from the trees. A wren hopping around in the mossy roots. Treecreepers creeping. Songbirds singing.

I spot different tawny owl couples, one handing over food from one partner to the other. Another day, the unmistakeable squeak of owlets calling to each other and their parents from the woods.

By mid-month, the sky is just starting to redden at the base of Dunmail Raise at 10.20pm.

It throws me into confusion every year when we seem to go straight from three-jumper weather to high summer, but it always seems to happen this way. It is bitterly cold, and then suddenly, it is warm and gentle.

The lake is delightfully inviting, the light soft and the air mild, teeming with bugs, keeping the swifts and martins and flycatchers and bats busy and happy.

I shed my socks, if I haven't already, then my gloves. It is so good to be released from them. To feel the water on my hands and toes again. To not have their wet weight to carry home.

I bring a book to the lake, lie in the sun after swimming and read, listening to the birds, distracted by watching damselflies rest and flit, rest and flit.

The bluebells peak and go over. After-work swims with friends extend to forgetting to go home for dinner. The light is so glorious and so long, the lake such easy company.

The badgers are frolicking in a pink glow at 10pm when I pass them on the walk home. The swimming year turns, flows on, is parted and rejoins itself. I travel over and through it. I let it carry me downstream. I let it take my weight.

May (again)

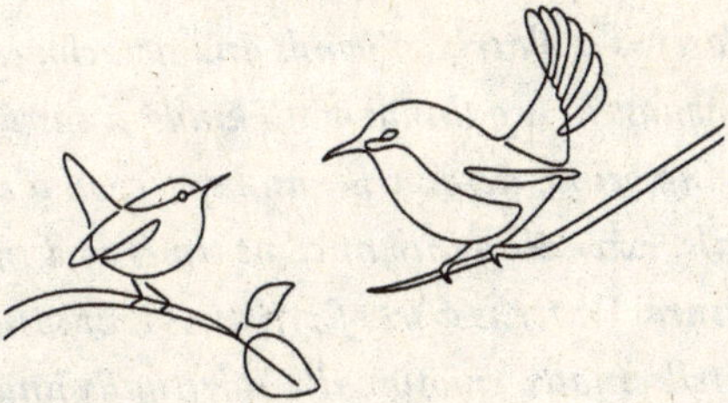

Water is a matrix of bonds and attachments amongst living things of all kinds, a cascade of living beings across time and space, on a cosmic scale, extending into ancient times and into the future. Water is a set of practices that socially, intellectually, emotionally, spiritually and physically reproduce the planet. Practices that are deeply relational and reciprocal. Practices that embody ethics privileging kindness and gentleness, creating architectures of care across time, space and species.

—Leanne Betasamosake Simpson,
Theory of Water

What to Wear

What should you wear to swim? A bikini, a one piece or shorts, a full wetsuit, nothing at all, or something in between? Only you can work out what works best for you, or what is possible, but it may take some trial and error to get it right.

Because what I want from swimming is swimming itself, it is more important to me to be as comfortable and safe in the water as I can be than to gain anything else from it. I am not convinced by any notion of biohacking or interested in self-discipline or achievement. This dictates not only how and when and where I swim, but what I wear when I'm swimming. I want to be able to swim as comfortably as possible, whatever the weather, whatever the season.

I lived here for over ten years as a summer swimmer. My swimming season ran from the first hot day in May to the last hot day in September, at best. Each autumn, I reluctantly bought a pass to one of the hotel pools in the village and brought my swimming indoors for the dark months.

Back then, I only knew a few people locally who swam outdoors all year round, all outliers in their own ways – all men, who swam naked, and took for granted a hardiness I knew I would never share. For many years, they would be the only people I would regularly see swimming on anything but the hottest summer days. I was the only one in a swimming costume, and felt overdressed.

I had been told the legend of Sally Woodhead when I first moved to Grasmere, a poet who had found refuge from the wider world at the Wordsworth Trust, like so many others. She had lived in the front room of Lake Terrace Two until her death, shortly before I arrived in Town End. I was told how she swam naked in Rydal Water every morning of the summer months regardless of the weather. How tough she was. How she rescued another staff member who got into trouble, underestimating the lake and overestimating his own fitness.

I admit I scoffed a little back then at the few wet-suited swimmers I would see in the summer. It seemed akin to turning up in a brand-new Range Rover – something for city folk on holiday, not locals – out of our price range and somehow showy.

Little by little, more people began to appear in our favoured spots, people who hadn't found them by word of mouth. Once, I arrived at a river pool that had been a local secret, and found a naked couple happily sunbathing on the pebbly beach.

I'd not seen them before, and as we chatted, I discovered they'd read about the spot in a guidebook. Over the following years, the occasional couple would become a steady trickle, and soon enough a torrent, bringing with them rubbish and barbecue burns and abandoned items of clothing. Not all the people, of course. But too many of them, careless in their own pleasure, as people so often are.

Down at the lake, more people in wetsuits began to appear throughout the year, trailing tow floats, though I didn't know they were called that then. The epoch of wild swimming had begun.

All this time, I kept expecting to acclimatise to the cold: that one day, I would find I could just stride into the lake and start swimming without wincing. But as the years passed, I seemed to find the cold harder, not easier. I wanted to keep swimming outdoors through the winter, but I could not see an eventuality where I would ever be able to just jump in as the winter swimmers I knew did.

I did not know why I struggled so much with the cold, only that I did. I didn't understand how I could want to swim so much but find the cold water so unbearable. I thought I wasn't doing enough to get stronger or braver.

Now I know it is a product of the connective tissue disorder I live with, and for many years was exacerbated by the blood-thickening effects of an untreated iron-loading disorder. After my diagnoses in my mid-thirties, I learnt to manage these conditions and their many symptoms and side-effects as best as I can. I learnt that my body cannot regulate itself to account for changing temperature, or move blood around itself efficiently. I learnt that this is why when I get cold, I keep getting colder, until I feel that my bones have been removed and replaced with ice. It explained why it takes so small a temperature drop for the blood to retreat from my fingers, toes and nose. It made sense of the many shapes and forms of pain cold brings me, my tendency towards chilblains, my delayed afterdrop. I had found through practice that I needed to keep moving in the water – the strategy I used to share with others as *Be A Shark!* Sharks die if they stop swimming, I would say. Keep swimming, and you'll be fine. *SHARK IT!* I would shout, as I swam in fast circles. Not all sharks need to keep moving to breathe like that, though, only certain species, and not all people need to keep moving so much in the water either. Many of my friends who swim all year are baskers who like to float, ottering, relishing the tingly feeling of cold on their skin, as I power past them counting breaths until I have acclimatised enough to relax.

Diagnosis also helped me begin to understand why I did not experience the cold thrill that other outdoor swimmers described: a euphoria catalysed by the meeting of cold water and the nervous system. No matter how cold the water, I felt no dopamine rush, so sudden sense of invulnerability or clarity. For so many years, I thought I was doing cold water wrong, that it wasn't cold enough or I wasn't in it enough, but it was my body doing things differently, as usual. I realised I needed to start doing things differently to work with my body and stop fighting against it.

In the autumn of 2017, I bought a shortie wet-suit – a surfing springsuit – in a sale. With long sleeves and short legs, it was easy enough to get on and off, not too heavy to carry, and allowed me to move my limbs freely in the water. It made it so much easier and more comfortable to get in on cooler days. I was less reliant on the sun to warm me, and less averse to the wind. With my shoulders and back insulated, I could stay in the cooling water long enough to swim, even if just for a short time. It is swimming I wanted, not just immersion. Without the legendary cold rush, a dip in and of itself did not mean much to me. I wanted to be able to move in the water safely. I wanted that release from gravity, that sense of being held and supported.

I swam until late November that way that year – amazed and delighted to keep the lake in my year so long. Though I stopped swimming over winter, I was back in the lake in April. I had extended my swimming year by over a month either end.

In autumn 2018, I got a small writing grant, and as I was partly writing about swimming, I set aside a little of it to buy a swimming wetsuit, and neoprene socks and gloves. That year, I swam through the winter for the first time.

Now, many seasons of swimming on, I know what I can tolerate better, what I can't, and how to work with it. I've learnt that a cold wind across the lake on a grey but mildish midwinter day is far more painful to me than a still, bright day below freezing. Cold wind is far worse than cold water, if there is sun on your face to change in.

Not everyone needs a wetsuit to swim through winter. I know many people who swim all year in ordinary swimwear – or none at all – sometimes with the addition of neoprene socks and gloves, sometimes just a woolly hat. Sometimes literally *just* a woolly hat. I'm told it's far easier this way – that you feel the cold less without wet kit to scrabble out of.

I wish I could swim all year without extra layers. They make swimming in winter possible for me, and for that I am grateful, but I don't like them, or the extra work they create. Like most people who live and work in the Lake District, I rent a home with an endemic damp problem: hardly the best environment for drying and maintaining human bodies in the winter months, let alone swimming kit. We lived for nine years with rain leaking intermittently into our bedroom before the roof was finally fixed. We don't have an outdoor tap for rinsing kit outside, and nowhere to hang it inside where it could plausibly dry overnight, even with a dehumidifier running. There's good reason hotels in the lakes have designated drying rooms. Our homes don't, though. Through winter, I am always trying and failing to dry out my socks and gloves before I want to use them again.

My conditions make managing the cold difficult, but they also make managing a wetsuit difficult. I have to be very careful not to pull shoulders and fingers out of joint putting a wetsuit on and off, and lack of sensation in my fingertips makes it hard to wiggle into one without damaging it, and even harder to get out if my fingers are too cold. The clumsiness inbuilt to Ehlers Danlos means I have a high propensity to damage expensive kit in one way or another. Joint and muscle pain, compounded by fatigue, makes it hard for me to carry kit, especially once it is wet and heavy.

There are also financial and ethical issues with wetsuits and other specialised outdoor swimming gear. Like all specialised kit, it is expensive. Even more so if you buy something and find after a few wears that it doesn't really work for you. There are places that hire out wetsuits and many companies will also sell seconds, ex-display or ex-rental suits, but that is expensive enough for the average person if you don't know what will be comfortable or practical for you. Wetsuit sizing can be confusing, as they traditionally only get bigger with height, so if you're a short curvy person with unusually long arms, like me, you're a bit stuck for a good fit. There are bespoke wetsuit services, but these are even more expensive.

There are also environmental costs to wetsuit use. Traditional wetsuits rely on neoprene, the first synthetic rubber, which was developed in the 1930s. Neoprene has many important uses besides wetsuits for leisure activities, but it is manufactured using petrochemicals, produces toxic carcinogenic waste during production, and is neither biodegradable nor compostable. Wetsuits are also often hard to recycle due to the way different materials are bonded together in their manufacture, so although they are widely used by people who value nature and the outdoors, their production and life cycle contributes to climate crisis. According to Full Circle, it is estimated that over a million wetsuits go into landfill every year. The last decade has seen more awareness of this paradox, and more recycling programmes to prevent old wetsuits ending up in landfill, but recycling petroleum neoprene into changing mats does not solve the problems of its production. The 2024 documentary *The Big Sea* highlighted the environmental impact of neoprene production in the surfing industry, and has helped accelerate the discussion and production of rubber alternatives.

Limestone neoprene – once seen as an ecological alternative to petroleum-based neoprene – has its own environmental toll, though it is still a better alternative to petroleum-based neoprene. Some brands have been experimenting with natural rubbers, such as Yulex, for over a decade, although some users argue they may not offer a like-for-like replacement. Yamamoto – the Japanese company that pioneered limestone neoprene in the 1960s as a sustainable and better quality alternative to petroleum neoprene – has recently developed a biodegradable version called Terraprene, which claims to offer the same performance.

At the moment, I can't see a way I could swim all year without some kind of thermal insulation. I alternate between an update of my original surfing springsuit – with long sleeves, a back zip and short legs – and a two-piece wetsuit with a pullover top like a mock neck, and bottoms like leggings. They have a great range of movement, and don't pinch or pull on my delicate skin as well as being easier to get on and off than a full wetsuit. They are also lighter to carry both dry and wet than any wetsuit I've tried so far. You can wear them together or separate, and the top is a useful, easily packable extra layer. Both of these are made of limestone neoprene. For much of winter now, I wear just the top over a long-sleeved swimming costume, with socks and gloves, of course. I save the leggings for windy days, or days I think I might not be able to shark it in the water. But I'm increasingly aware of the wider implications of these layers I find essential to my enjoyment of the water.

Living in an age of climate crisis, especially as a disabled person, is to exist in continual compromise between physical needs and environmental impact. I don't want my relationship with the place I love to come at the cost of the place I love, nor of any other place either. I can't gaze at the fells and woods of the lakes and put out of mind distant landfill sites overflowing with the toxic detritus of western quests for wellbeing. I can't luxuriate in a sparkling upland river without remembering the rivers polluted by production of the kit that lets me be in it.

Maybe all we can do as individuals is try our best, do our research, and try and manage our waste responsibly. What we can do together to shift a culture of consumption might be much more impactful.

Maybe one day, I will be able to shed these layers. Through continued practice and careful management, I have begun to adjust just a sliver to the cold. But I am a long way from relishing it. I still wait all year for the few weeks in summer when I can swim without shivering, where I can go to the water as I used to, back when I first started swimming in the lakes: just me, a towel, a book, and a drink. When I can dry out in the sun, and be warm enough to get back in again if time and energy allows.

As a disabled person, I also know the things I take for granted now could change at any moment. I could find myself suddenly immured to the cold. I could find myself suddenly unable to swim at all. I could find the water too dangerous to swim in again.

For now, I try to keep what balance I can. To stay present, in my own way, with thought and care. To continue, in the ordinary and extraordinary ways of the chronically ill. To do what I can, when I can, for myself, for the places I love, for the network of community local and global that that love places me in. For the present, the past, the future.

Resources and Further Reading

The growth of interest in outdoor swimming has also given rise to a growth in books on swimming, from where-to and how-to guides, logbooks and journals, and swim-lit – swimming literature.

Outdoor Swimmer magazine is a great source of information on all things outdoor swimming, and has regular guidance on swimming gear and reviews of latest developments in wetsuits, goggles, changing robes and more. It's a beautiful and informative magazine whatever kind of swimming you do. It also runs courses, including an online course on preparing for winter swimming.

Some guides to outdoor swimming that give useful advice on preparation and kit:

How to Wild Swim: What to Know Before Taking the Plunge by Ella Foote (Dorling Kindersley, 2023)

The Outdoor Swimmers' Handbook by Kate Rew (Rider, 2022)

Swim Wild and Free: A Practical Guide to Swimming Outdoors 365 Days a Year by Simon Griffiths (Bloomsbury Sport, 2022)

Swimming Wild in the Lake District by Suzanna Cruickshank (Vertebrate, 2020) (Suzanna is also an excellent swim guide you can book for individual or group sessions.)

If you're looking for more descriptive accounts of swimming, these are some non-fiction books that centre swimming that I've particularly enjoyed and often recommend:

Swims by Elizabeth Jane Burnett (Penned in the Margins, 2017)

Turning by Jessica J. Lee (Virago, 2017)

Why We Swim by Bonnie Tsui (Rider, 2021)

Swimming Studies by Leanne Shapton (Particular Books, 2012)

The Tidal Year by Freya Bromley (Coronet, 2023)

At the Pond: Swimming at the Hampstead Ladies' Pond, various (Daunt, 2019)

By the River: Essays from the Water's Edge, various (Daunt, 2024)

Swimming With Seals by Victoria Whitworth (Apollo, 2021)

Small Bodies of Water by Nina Mingya Powles (Canongate, 2022)

The Outrun by Amy Liptrot (Canongate, 2015)

The Apothecary by the Sea by Victoria Bennett (Elliott and Thompson, 2026)

Shorelines by Alycia Pirmohamed (Canongate, 2026)

My Body is a Meadow by Bethany Handley (Headline, 2026)

Books on water and bodies of water more generally I recommend include:

Theory of Water: Nishnaabe Maps to the Times Ahead by Leanne Betasamosake Simpson (Haymarket, 2025)

The Flow by Amy-Jane Beer (Bloomsbury Wildlife, 2023)

Is a River Alive? by Robert Macfarlane (Hamish Hamilton, 2025)

How to Read Water by Tristan Gooley (Hodder, 2017)

A Barrister for the Earth by Mónica Feria-Tinta (Faber and Faber, 2025)

Thirst: In Search of Freshwater, various (Wellcome Collection, 2025)

Sea Bean by Sally Huband (Penguin, 2024)

For more information on freshwater water biosecurity, see West Cumbria Rivers Trust: https://www.westcumbriariverstrust.org/dont-pack-a-pest

Endnotes

1 https://www.westcumbriariverstrust.org/wildlife/inns

2 https://www.savewindermere.com/

3 https://www.thewestmorlandgazette.co.uk/news/238995.clean-up-for-grasmere/

4 https://www.thewestmorlandgazette.co.uk/news/6924955.grasmere-clean-up-begins/

5 https://www.cnp.org.uk/our-national-parks/why-we-campaign/nature/water/

Acknowledgements

With thanks to everyone who has encouraged me to swim, swum alongside me or waited patiently by the shore. Especially my mum, who wanted to make sure I had the confidence in the water she never did.

Extracts from Alycia Pirmohamed, Elizabeth-Jane Burnett, Bethany Handley, Jessica J. Lee, Clare Shaw, Emily Hasler, Nina Mingya Powles, Bonnie Tsui and Leanne Betasamosake Simpson quoted with kind permission of the authors and/or their publishers. Rose Macaulay quoted with kind permission of The Society of Authors as the Literary Representative of the Estate of Rose Macaulay.

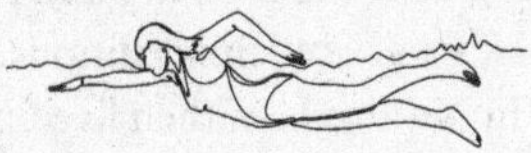

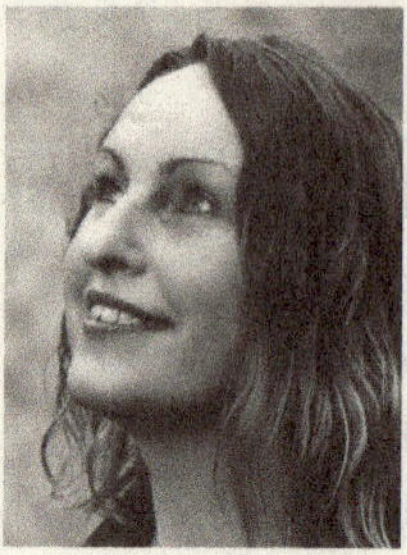

Polly Atkin (FRSL) is a poet and nonfiction writer whose work focuses on nature, place and disability. Her poetry collections are *Basic Nest Architecture* (Seren: 2017), *Much With Body* (Seren: 2021) and *Emergency Dream* (Seren: 2026). *Recovering Dorothy: The Hidden Life of Dorothy Wordsworth* (Saraband: 2021), the first biography of Dorothy Wordsworth's later life and illness, was longlisted for the Barbellion Prize 2022. Her memoir *Some Of Us Just Fall: On Nature and Not Getting Better* (Sceptre: 2023 and Unnamed: 2024)) was named Lakeland Book of the Year 2024 and longlisted for the Wainwright Prize for Nature Writing 2024. Her third nonfiction book *The Company of Owls* (Elliott and Thompson: 2024 and Milkweed: 2026) was longlisted for the Wainwright Prize for Nature Writing 2025. Her poetry and prose appears in various anthologies and academic editions.

She grew up in Nottingham then lived in East London for seven years before moving north to Cumbria. She has a PhD from Lancaster University and taught English and Creative Writing at QMUL, Lancaster University, and the Universities of Strathclyde and Cumbria. She works as a freelancer from her home in the English Lake District, where she co-owns historic Grasmere bookshop Sam Read Bookseller.